ECG MADE EASY
HOT NOTES BY Dr. M.O.H.M.

2021

ECG MADE EASY : HOT NOTES BY Dr. M.O.H.M.

Contents:

INTRODUCTION	2
WAVES & INTERVALS	6
CARDIAC AXIS	10
HYPERTROPHY	12
ISCHEMIC HEART DISEASE	13
HEART BLOCK	15
DYSARRHYTHMIA	17
HYPERKALEMIA & HYPOKALEMIA	20
PERICARDITIS VS. INFARCTION	21
HOW TO READ & REPORT THE ECG	22
OTHER TOPICS	23

ECG by M.O.H.M — INTRODUCTION

ECG by M.O.M – INTRODUCTION

In this chapter, I would like to explain some practical points in the *basics of the ECG interpretation*.. and answer the two important questions..
' *HOW TO READ THE ECG ?* ' &
' *HOW TO REPORT THE ECG ?* '..

So, by the end of this chapter you should have a systematic approach to interpreting the ECG and be able to identify the common ECG abnormalities.

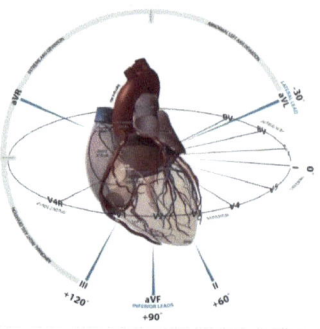
www.lifeinthefastlane.com

The 12 lead ECG:

The 12 lead ECG is made up of the three standard limb leads (I, II and III), the augmented limb leads (aVR, aVL and aVF) and the six precordial leads (V1, V2, V3, V4, V5 and V6).

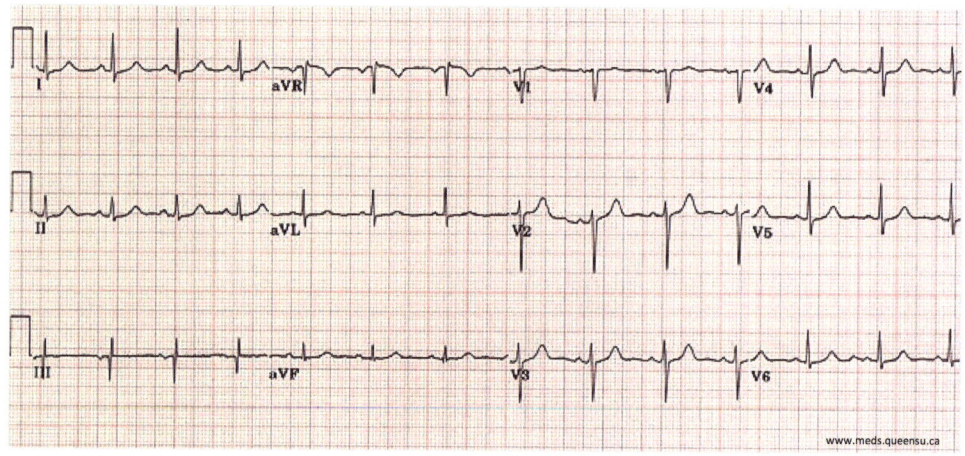

A normal ECG is illustrated above. Note that the heart is beating in a regular sinus rhythm between 60 - 100 beats per minute (specifically 82 bpm). All the important intervals on this recording are within normal ranges.

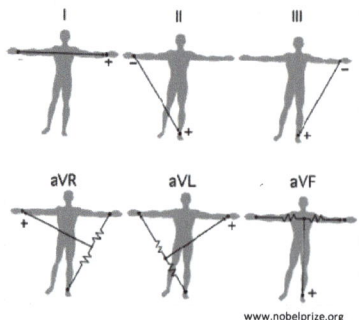
www.nobelprize.org

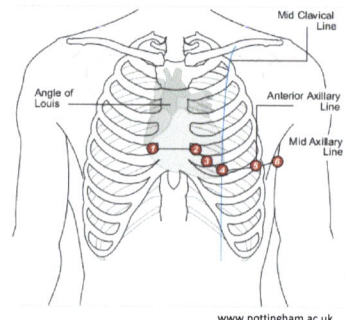
www.nottingham.ac.uk

ECG by M.O.H.M — INTRODUCTION..

Trick: *NEVER FORGET THIS TOPIC..*

Localization of the abnormality:

the directions from which the various leads look at the heart:

- V1-V4   anteroseptal wall
- V5-V6   lateral wall

   V1-V2   septal wall
   V3-V4   anterior wall
   V5-V6   lateral wall

- II, III, aVF   inferior wall
- I, aVL   lateral wall
- V1-V2   posterior wall *(reciprocal)*

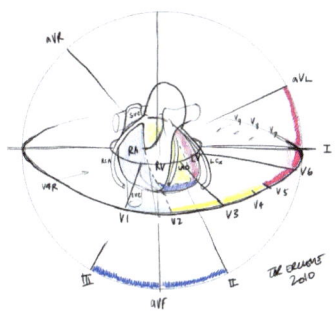

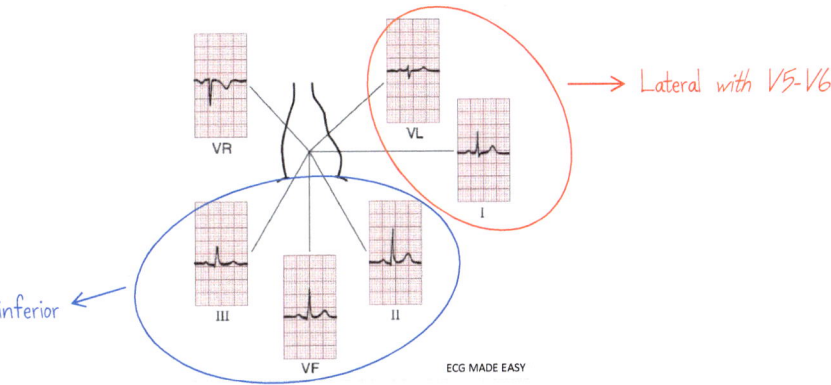

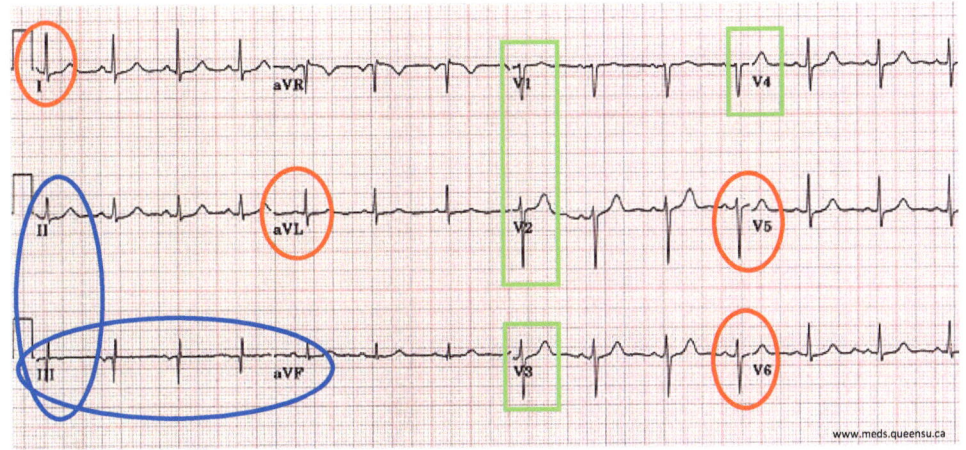

ECG MADE EASY : HOT NOTES BY Dr. M.O.H.M.

ECG by M.O.H.M — INTRODUCTION..

ECG thermal paper:

the ECG paper consists from large (▢) & small (▫) squares.. the relationship between the squares on ECG paper, time & voltage is explained in the figure below:

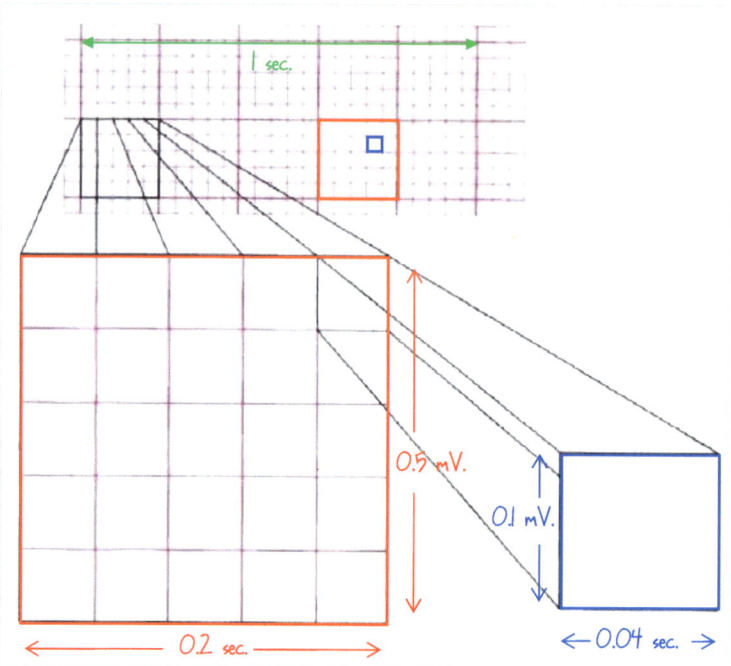

www.scribd.com – understanding ECG

Calibration & Speed:

it is important to make sure normal calibration & speed in every ECG..

normal calibration = 1mV. = 1cm. &

normal speed = 25 mm./sec..

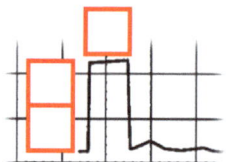

Trick: so, 2 large squares X 1 large square is a must..

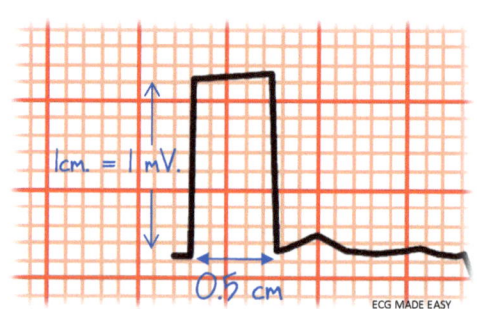

ECG MADE EASY

ECG by M.O.H.M — INTRODUCTION..

Heart rate:

The ideal way to calculate the heart rate is by count the no. of *small* or *large* squares between the 2 consecutive R waves, then calculate the heart rate by one of these equations:

Heart rate = 1500 / no. of R-R ☐   or   Heart rate = 300 / no. of R-R ☐

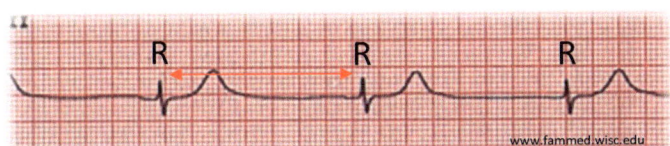

Count number of large boxes between first and second R waves = 7.5 .. 300/7.5 large boxes = rate 40

★★ You can use S wave as well..

Trick: The practical way to calculate the rate is depend on the no. of large squares between 2 consecutive R waves and as the following..

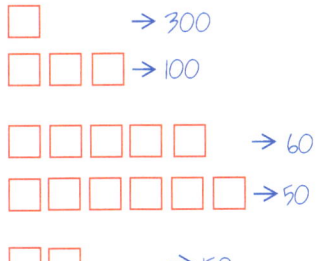

☐ → 300
☐☐ → 100
☐☐☐☐ → 60
☐☐☐☐☐ → 50
☐☐ → 150
☐☐☐☐ → 75

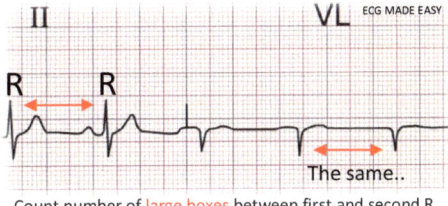

Count number of large boxes between first and second R waves = 4 .. So, the heart rate = 75

if you have an *irregular rhythm* (like atrial fibrillation).. so, when you want to know an average rate, you can use the six-second method:

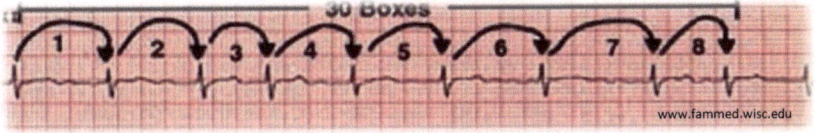

Count 30 large boxes, starting from the first R wave. There are 8 R-R intervals within 30 boxes. Multiply 8 × 10 = Rate 80.

ECG by M.O.H.M — WAVES & INTERVALS..

Waves & intervals:

The picture of an ECG consists of several waves, complexes, intervals & segments..
So, I would like to explain each of these components individually..
BUT, first you have to know some of their definitions and general idea to be oriented... :

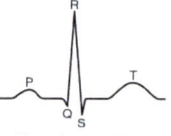

Waves & complexes:

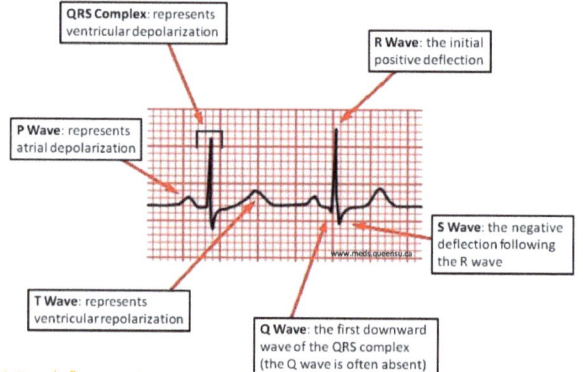

- **QRS Complex**: represents ventricular depolarization
- **R Wave**: the initial positive deflection
- **P Wave**: represents atrial depolarization
- **S Wave**: the negative deflection following the R wave
- **T Wave**: represents ventricular repolarization
- **Q Wave**: the first downward wave of the QRS complex (the Q wave is often absent)

Intervals & segments:

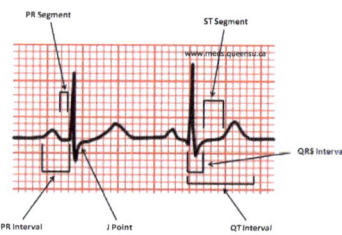

PR Interval:	From the start of the P wave to the start of the QRS complex
PR Segment:	From the end of the P wave to the start of the QRS complex
J Point:	The junction between the QRS complex and the ST segment
QT Interval:	From the start of the QRS complex to the end of the T wave
QRS Interval:	From the start to the end of the QRS complex
ST Segment:	From the end of the QRS complex (J point) to the start of the T wave

WAVES & INTERVALS..

Trick: no. of □ X 0.04 = time in seconds..

P wave:

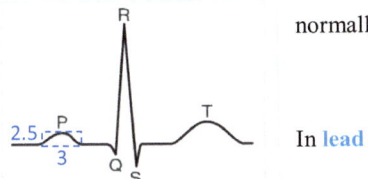

normally: 3□ X 2.5□

+ve except in (aVR –ve)

In lead I : almost always +ve..
If –ve → either *wrong connection* or *dextrocardi*

In left atrium enlargement: *bifid P* wave in leads I, aVL, may be II
biphasic in V_1

In right atrium enlargement: *tented P wave* in leads II, III, aVF & V_1

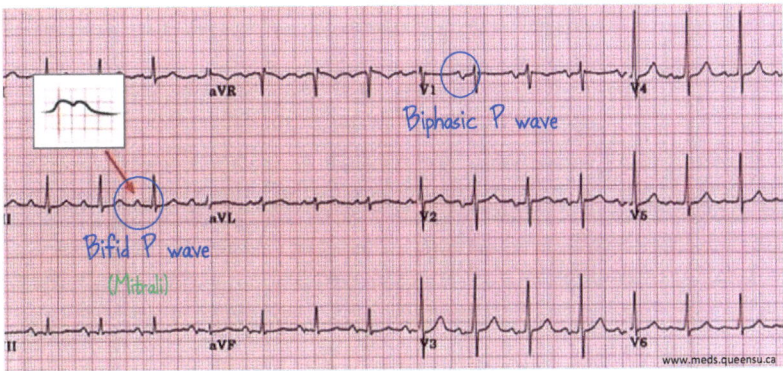

Left atrial enlargement: the P wave in lead II is bifid & the P wave in lead V_1 is biphasic (has terminal negative deflection)..

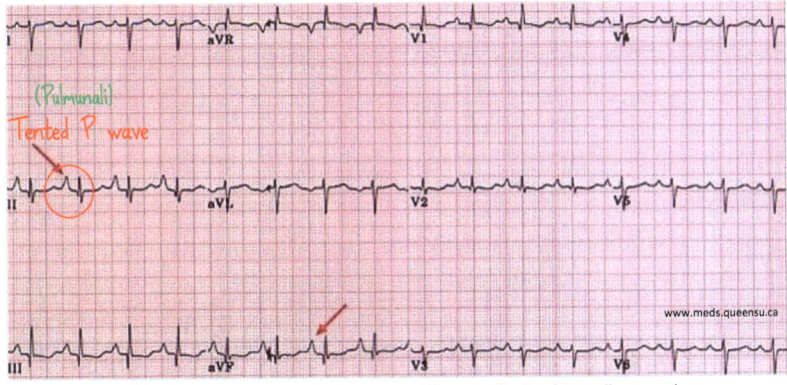

Right atrial enlargement: the P wave in lead II is tented (has amplitude of 4 small squares)..

ECG by M.O.H.M — WAVES & INTERVALS..

P-R interval:

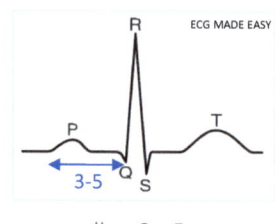

normally = 3 – 5 □

QRS complex:

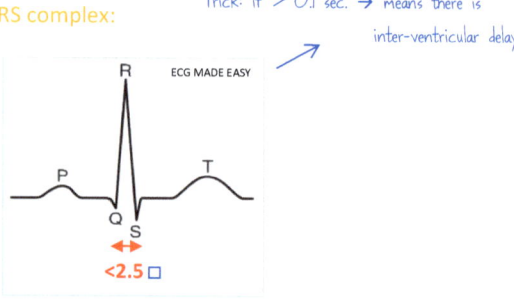

<2.5 □

normally = (0.06-0.1 sec.)

Trick: if > 0.1 sec. → means there is inter-ventricular delay..

Q wave:

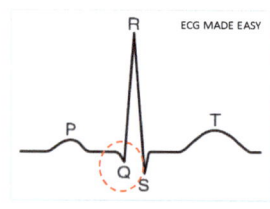

normally in aVR..

normal *septal Q* wave → < 25% of R wave
        < □ (0.04 sec.)

pathological Q wave → > 25% of R wave or
        > □ (0.04 sec.)

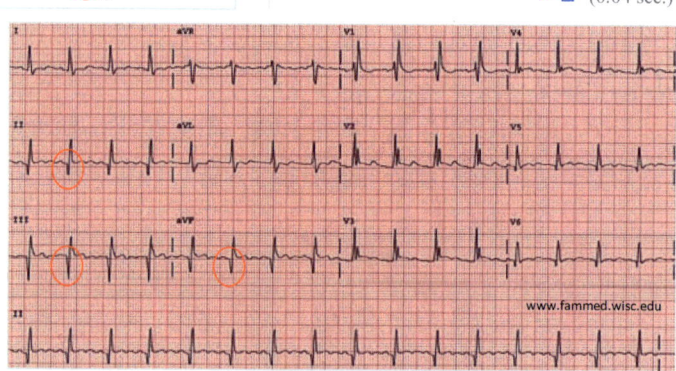

Note *pathological Q waves* in leads II, III, and aVF (inferior wall infarction)..

ST segment:

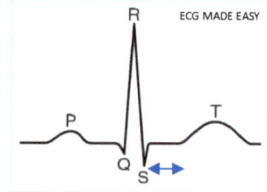

normally is isoelectrical..

abnormal → *elevation*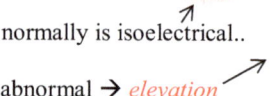
   in (M.I or pericarditis)

or *depression*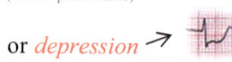
   in (ischemia, electrolyte disturbances, ventricular hypertrophy)

T wave:

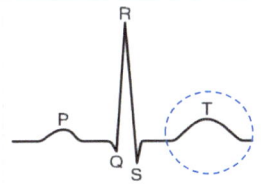

normally: +ve in leads I, II, V$_{3-6}$

inverted in aVR

variable in the other leads

normal height → *5 mm.* in *limb* leads (one ☐)

10 mm. in *chest leads* (two ☐)

more than this range it is consider as a *tall, tented T wave*.. like in: M.I, ↑K⁺, C.V.A..

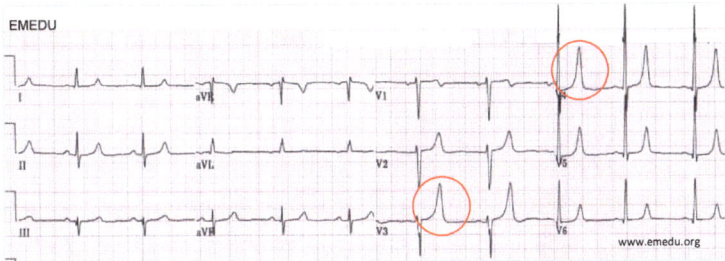

Hyperkalemia: Note the *tall, tented T waves*..

QT interval:

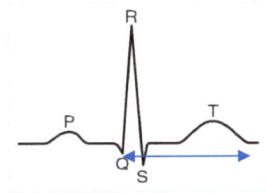

normally : 8 – 11.5 ☐ (0.32 – 0.46 sec.)
prolonged in → heart failure, ↓Ca^{+2}, drugs

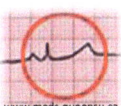

U wave:

is a small (0.5 mm) deflection *immediately following the T wave*, usually in the same direction as the T wave, may be normal in ECG, especially in V$_3$..

prominant in ↓K⁺ & opposite to T wave in myocardial ischemia..

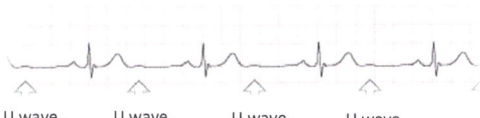

U wave..   U wave..   U wave..   U wave..

ECG by M.O.H.M — THE CARDIAC AXIS..

Calculation of the electrical axis:

The mean QRS axis refers to the average orientation of the heart's electrical activity. In most cases, an approximation of the axis will be sufficient for the ECG interpretation. There are many different approaches to axis determination, but this discussion will be limited to two approaches only ' *the practical & ideal approaches* '..

Trick:

The practical approaches: is depends on the QRS deflection in the leasds I, II, III..

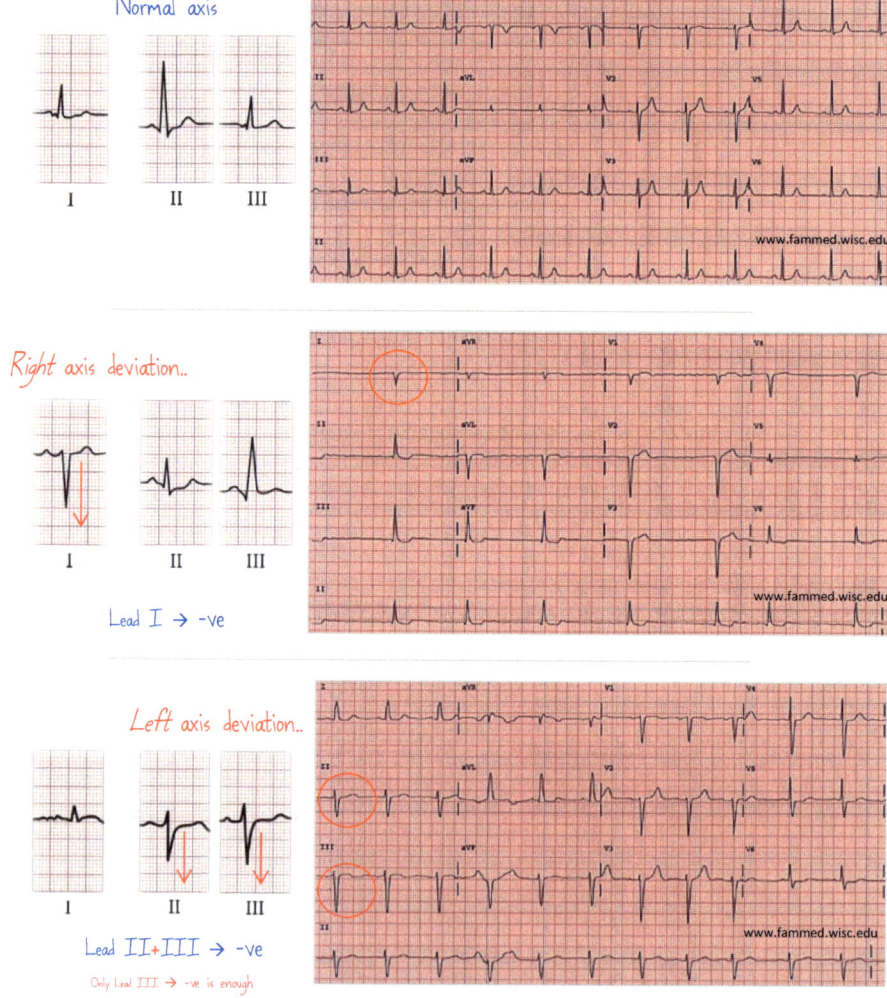

Normal axis
I   II   III

Right axis deviation..
I   II   III
Lead I → -ve

Left axis deviation..
I   II   III
Lead II+III → -ve
Only Lead III → -ve is enough

ECG by M.O.H.M — THE CARDIAC AXIS..

The *ideal* approach:

The mean QRS axis is oriented towards the lead with the greatest net QRS deflection. To calculate the net QRS deflection, add up the number of small squares that correspond to the height of the R wave (positive deflection), and subtract the number of small squares that correspond to the height of the Q and S waves (negative deflection).

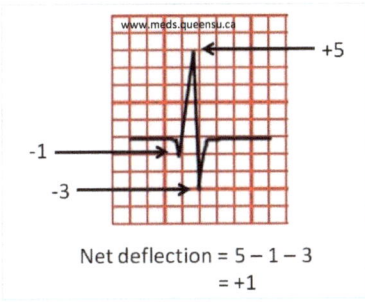

Approximate the net QRS deflection for leads I and aVF. Remember that the mean QRS axis will be oriented towards the lead with the greatest positive net QRS deflection. If the net deflection is positive for both, the axis lies between leads I and aVF (0-90°) and is therefore normal.

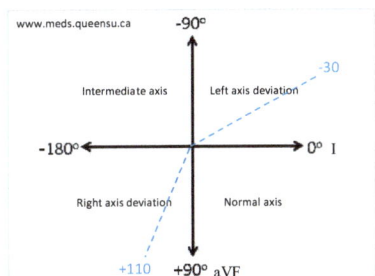

You have to remember this image to use this approach..

For example..

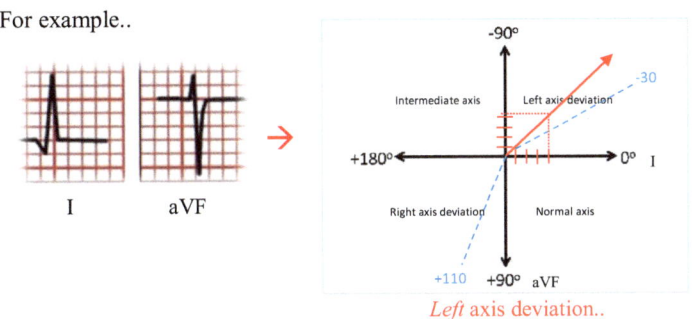

Left axis deviation..

ECG by M.O.H.M — HYPERTROPHY..

Ventricular hypertrophy:

Left ventricular hypertrophy (L.V.H.):

If.. The S wave in V_1
+
The R wave in $V_{5\,or\,6}$

Note: if the L.V.H. is *sever*, you will see ST depression and T wave inversion in the lateral leads I, aVL & V_{5-6}.

> 35 □ → L.V.H.

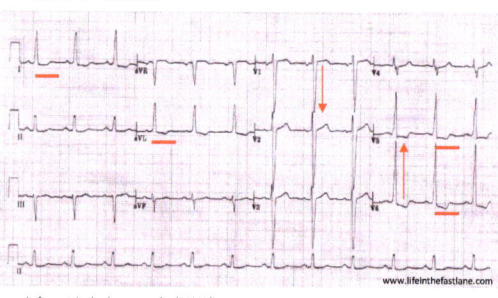

Left ventricular hypertrophy (L.V.H.)..

Right ventricular hypertrophy (R.V.H.):

If.. The R ≥ S wave in V_1
The S ≥ R wave in V_6

Note: if the R.V.H. is *sever*, you will see ST depression &T wave inversion in the V_{2-3} due to hypertrophy (not M.I.)..

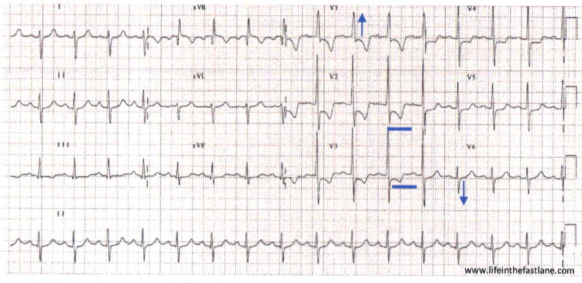

Right ventricular hypertrophy (R.V.H.)..

Ischemic heart disease:

Angina pectoris:

Only 50% of cases get ECG changes..

The ECG abnormality is **ST depression** except in *prinzmetal angina* (***ST elevation***).

Myocardial infarction:

It is either *ST elevation myocardial infarction* (**STEMI**) or *non-ST elevation myocardial infarction* (**non-STEMI** ' the ST segment is isoelectrical with T wave inversion ')..

Timing:

Acute M.I → ST elevation, hyper-acute T wave..

Recent M.I → ST elevation, T wave inversion..

Old M.I → only Q wave..

Localization: Please, see page 39... & **NEVER** forget it...

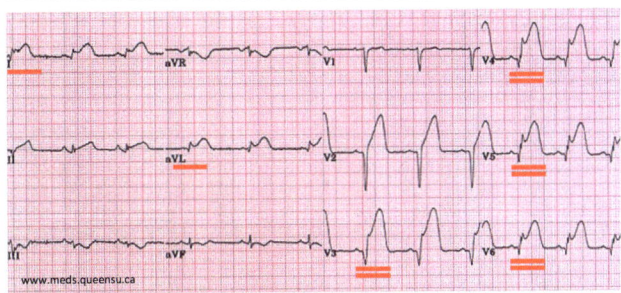

Acute Antero-lateral M.I.

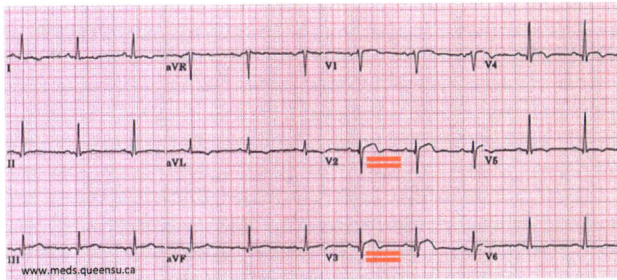

Acute Septal M.I.

ISCHEMIC HEART DISEASE..

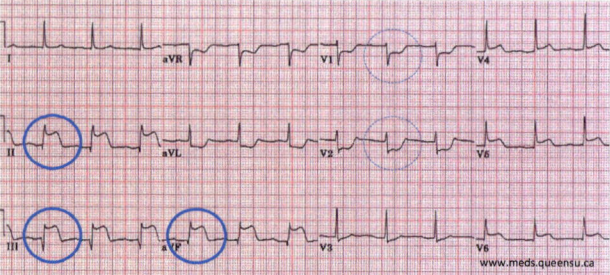

Acute Inferior M.I. associated with ' posterior infarction.. ST segments in leads overlying the posterior region of the heart (V1 and V2) are initially horizontally depressed. As the infarction evolves, lead V1 demonstrates an R wave (which in fact represents a Q wave in reverse).. '

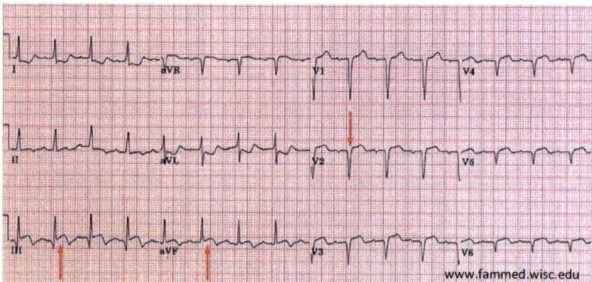

The pathological Q waves seen in V1 - V6 indicate that this patient has had an anterior MI in the past. This patient also has evidence of an acute inferior MI as shown by the ST segment elevation in leads III and aVF.

Heart block:

Atrioventricular block:

1st degree:

P wave & QRS complex → normal

PR interval → prolonged (> 5□) (> 0.2 sec.)

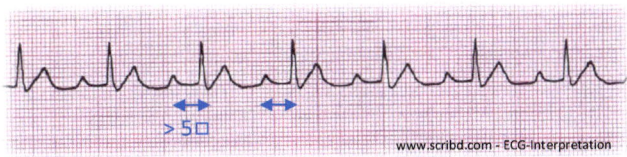

2nd degree:

1- Morbitz type 1: *'Wenckeback phenomena'*

Progressive PR prolongation then dropped QRS..

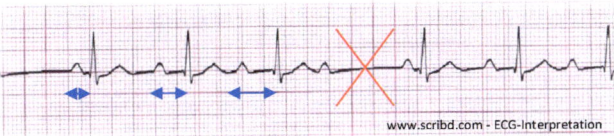

2- Morbitz type 2:

Sudden drop of QRS, without prior PR changes..

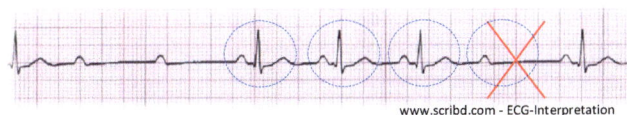

3rd degree:

P is not related to QRS.. PP rate is regular, BUT is differ from the RR rate (which is also regular)..

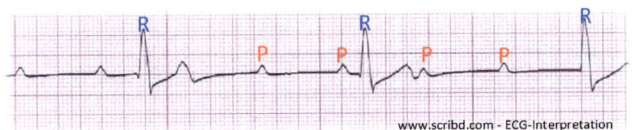

ECG by M.O.H.M — HEART BLOCK..

Note:
The QRS complex in the chest leads shows a ***progression*** from lead V_1, where it is predominantly *downward*, to lead V_6, where it is predominantly *upward*. The ' transition point ', where the R & S waves are equal, indicates the position of the interventricular septum. So, if the right ventricle is enlarged, and occupies more of the precordium than is normal, the transition point will move from its normal position of leads V_3/V_4 to leads V_4/V_5 or sometimes leads V_5/V_6.

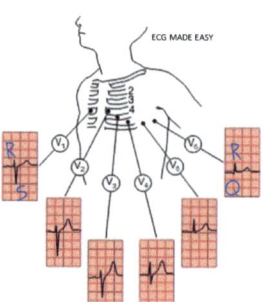

Trick:
You have to know, there is R & S waves in the lead V_1 BUT Q & S waves in V_6 (which is normal septal Q wave) → So, any change in this figure, think about any abnormality like Bundle branch block..

Right bundle branch block (RBBB):
QRS > 0.12 (> 3 □)
In the.. lead V_1 → RSR' wave *(M shape)*.. leads I & V_6 → *slurred ' broad ' S wave*
leads V_{1-3} → T wave inversion
causes : ***Idiopathic***, 2° to COPD or 2° to right ventricular pressure overload.

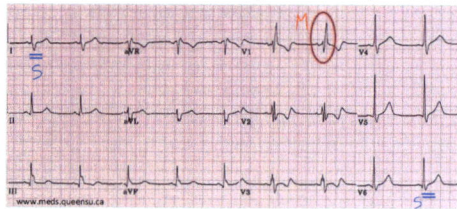

Left bundle branch block (RBBB):
QRS > 0.11 (> 3 □)
In the.. lead I, aVL & V_{5-6} → RSR' wave *(M shape)* and ST depression & T inversion
causes : acute M.I, sever L.V.H., sever aortic stenosis, cardiomyopathy & rarely ***Idiopathic***.

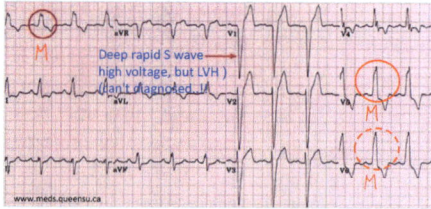

Dysarrhythmia:

We depend on the *lead II* strip.. & you have to observe the following:
the rate is *regular, regular irregular, irregular irregular..?*
the P wave & its relation to QRS..
P wave & QRS complex configuration..

Sinus rhythm:
There is P wave for each QRS complex..

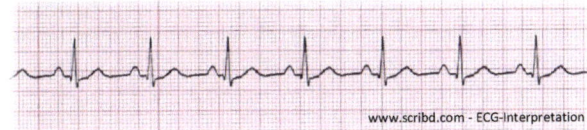

Sinus bradycardia:
P wave for each QRS
PP rate & RR rate *< 60* beats/minute
Causes : athletes, hypothyroidism, hypothermia, increase intracranial pressure & inferior M.I.

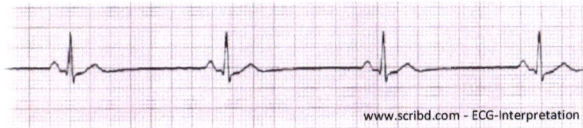

Sinus tachycardia:
P wave for each QRS
PP rate & RR rate *>100* beats/minute
Causes : fever, anxiety, exercise, anemia, hyperthyroidism..

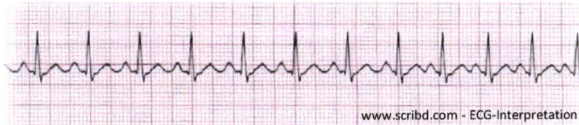

Sinus arrhythmia:
P wave for each QRS
when *longest RR > shortest RR* by *0.16 sec.* (4 □) then sinus arrhythmia is diagnosed..
Causes : normal in infant & young children.. pathological in elderly..

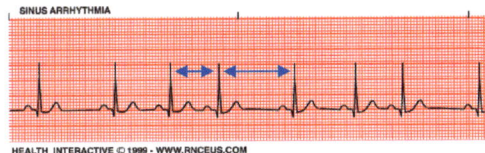

DYSARRHYTHMIA..

Atrial premature contraction (A.P.C.):
Normal ECG → P wave for each QRS
BUT, one P wave is different from previous one &
the PR interval in this beat is changeable..

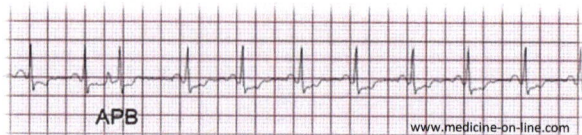

Ventricular premature beat (V.P.B.):
rate → regular
No P wave, *wide QRS*, *T wave is opposite* to QRS..
usually followed by compensatory pause..
could be single or multiple.

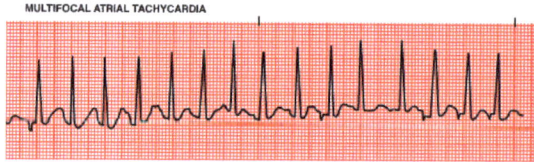

Multifocal atrial tachycardia:
Different *p wave*, *PR interval*, *PP & RR rate*..
multiple area of P wave origin.. & usually seen in advance pulmonary disease..

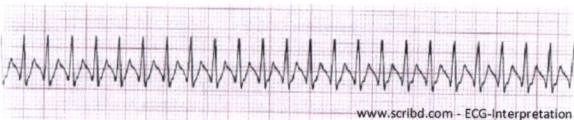

Supra-ventricular tachycardia (S.V.T.):
Heart rate = *160 – 220* b./min.
regular rhythm..

Atrial flutter:
Atrial rate = *250-350* b./min. regular..
PP rate faster than RR rate..
AV block: 2:1, 3:1, 4:1 … etc
ventricular rate is regular or irregular (depending on the degree of the block)..

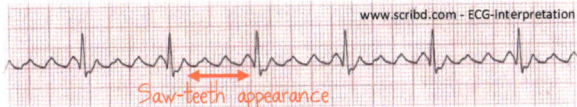

Atrial fibrillation:
rate → completely irregular *' irregular irregular '*..
No P wave, but there is **F wave** *' fibrillatory wave '*
Atrial rate = 350-450, ventricular rate is completely irregular..
there is two type of fibrillation: fine and coarse atrial fibrillation..

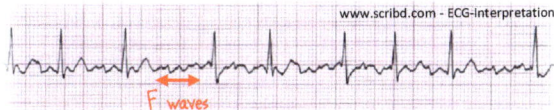

Ventricular tachycardia (V.T.):
No P wave, wide QRS complex, **fast tachycardia..**
usually serious dysarrhythmia → may progress to serious ventricular tachycardia..

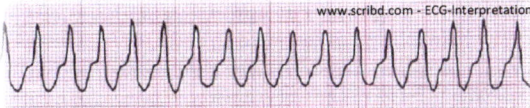

Trick:
Whenever you say *ventricular* beat, this is mean no P wave, wide QRS complex..

Ventricular fibrillation: ' FATAL DYSARRHYTHMIA '
No actual QRS.. rather *bizarre & chaotic undulation* of the base..
there is two type of ventricular fibrillation: fine and coarse fibrillation..

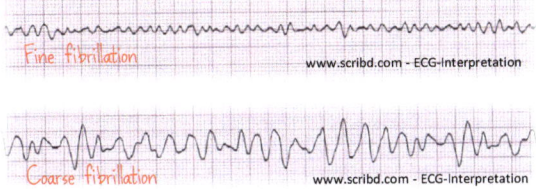

Hyperkalemia & hypokalemia:

Hyperkalemia:

There are *tall, tented, symmetrical T waves* with a narrow base..

The P wave remains normal, as does the QRS complex. the QRS complex broadens and the S wave is widened in leads V3 - V6. This S wave become continuous with the tented T waves and eventually the ST segment disappears.

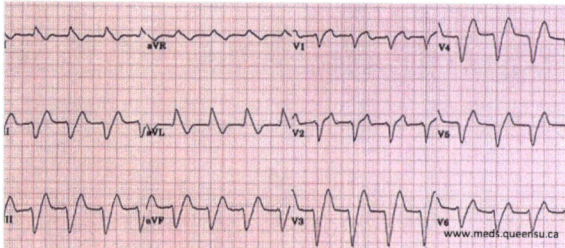

Hypokalemia:

There are *flattening of the T waves*, *U waves* may develop..

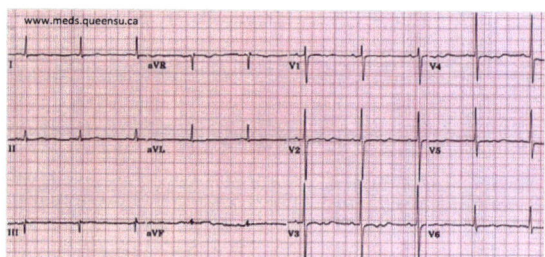

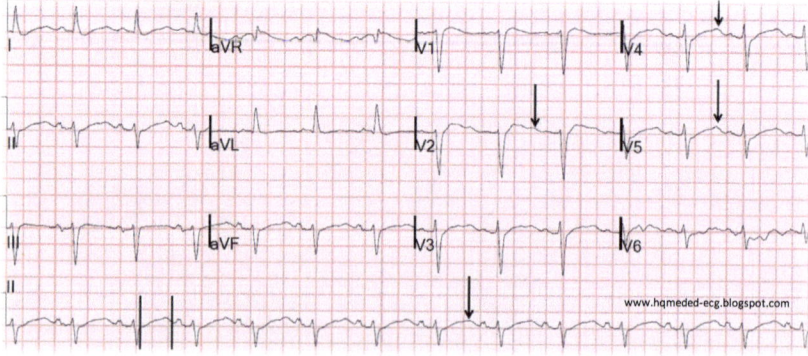

Notice large U-waves (arrows). One is tempted to think that the long hump after the QRS (between the two vertical lines) is the T-wave. Whenever you see this, you should think about both long QT and U-wave. But if you look closely, you see there are 2 bumps, so the second one must be a U-wave.

Pericarditis vs. Infarction:

Acute pericarditis:
ST segment *elevation, concave* upward....
Usually *diffused*
Start as ST segment elevation → back normal → T wave inversion
No reciprocal changes.. No pathological Q wave
May be PR segment depression '*very sensitive indicator of acute pericarditis* '..

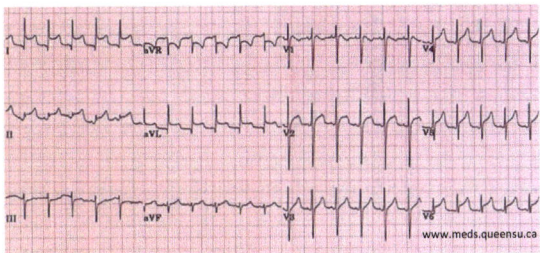

Myocardial infarction:
ST segment *elevation, convex* upward....
Usually *localized*
ST segment elevation, Q wave, T wave inversion may be together..
May be there is reciprocal changes..

Trick:
You can draw an imaginary line between the J point and the apex of the T wave. If the ST segment is below that line, then it's upwardly concave. If it's even with or above that line, then it's upwardly convex, which is suspicious for acute myocardial infarction.

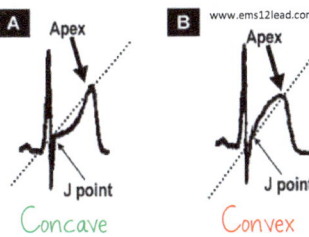

If it helps you to remember, an upwardly concave ST segment makes a "smiley face" (good) and an upwardly convex ST segment makes a "frowny face" (bad).

So, take it easy..
Dr. M.O.M

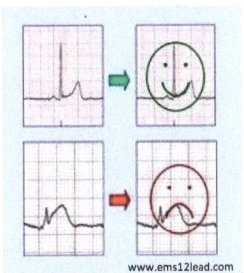

HOW TO READ & REPORT THE ECG??..

How to *read & report* the ECG ??

Answer:
It is a **matter of training**..

so, whenever you see an ECG.. read it *systematically* and don't put the diagnosis as an aim.. with time and when you become able to catch a lot of abnormalities then you can easily reach a possible diagnosis..

How to read the ECG ?

1- Start from the labeling.. (NAME, AGE, SEX, EXACT TIME)
2- See the calibration & speed..
3- Make sure normal connection & no dextrocardia

4- Rate & rhythm
5- Axis

6- P wave ' in leads I, II, V_1 '
7- PR interval ' in the lead II strip is the best '

8- QRS complexes & Q wave ' also look for ventricular hypertrophy & bundle branch block '
9- ST segment & T wave

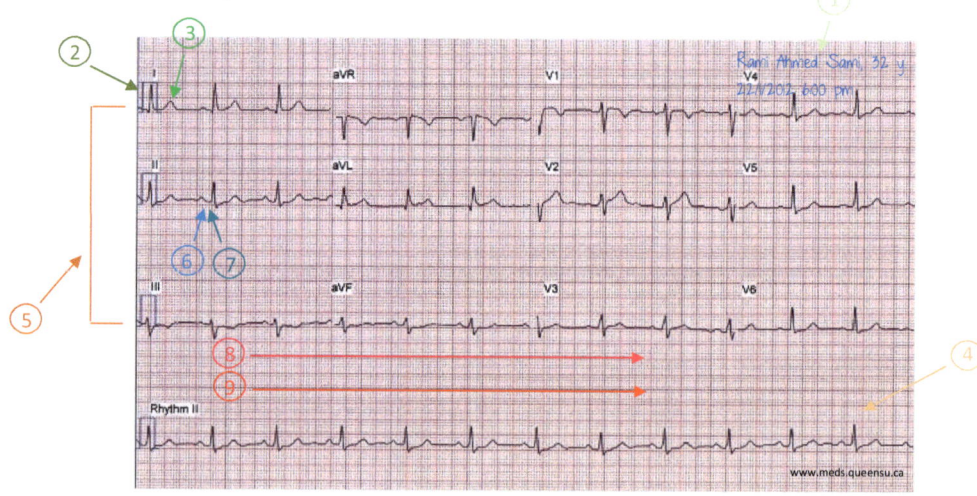

How to report the ECG ?

In the same sequence as for reading the ECG.. but, please don't mention the headlines.. So, *FORGET:*
the ~~NAME, AGE, SEX, EXACT TIME, ... RATE, RHYTHM~~.... etc.
just like in the reporting of the history..

ECG by M.O.H.M — OTHER TOPICS..

Inverted P wave in lead I:

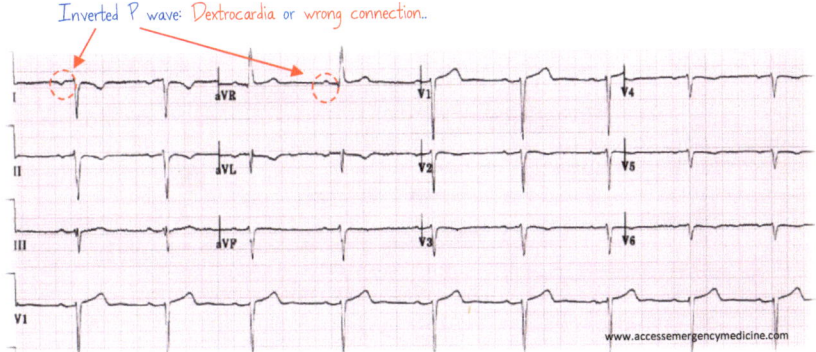

Inverted P wave: Dextrocardia or wrong connection..

Digoxin toxicity:

Digoxin effect refers to the presence on the ECG of:
Down-sloping ST depression with a characteristic *"sagging"* appearance
Flattened, inverted, or biphasic T waves.
Shortened QT interval

The morphology of the QRS complex / ST segment is variously described as either slurred, sagging or scooped and resembling either a reverse tick, hockey stick or (my personal favorite) **' Salvador Dali's moustache ' !**

The most common T-wave abnormality is a **biphasic T wave** with an initial negative deflection and terminal positive deflection. This is usually seen in leads with a dominant R wave (e.g. V4-6). The first part of the T wave is typically continuous with the depressed ST segment. The terminal positive deflection may be peaked, or have a prominent U wave superimposed upon it.

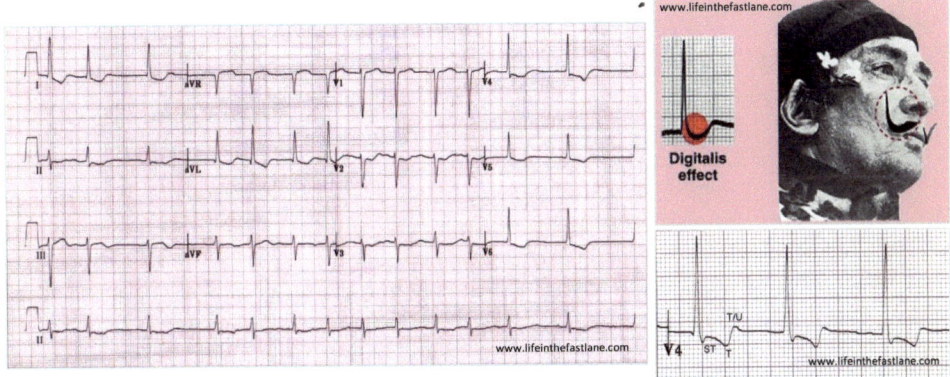

Wolff-Parkinson-White syndrome:

Diagnosis of W.P.W. is based on the ECG interpretation..

PR interval <0.12 seconds, P waves of normal appearance

QRS complex is wide, with a longer duration than 0.12 seconds

The presence of delta waves ' Slow enrollment or thickening of the initial portion of the QRS complex (delta wave) is the most important criterion for diagnosis of Wolff-Parkinson-White syndrome, Delta wave length range between 0.02-0.07 seconds '

Secondary changes of ST segment and T wave, which are showing a opposite direction from the QRS complex and delta wave.

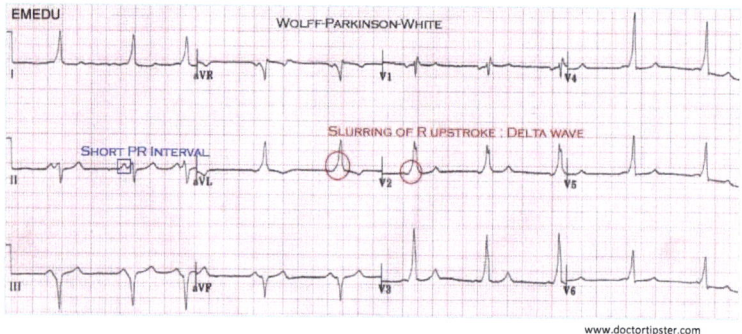

Ventricular asystole:

Simply, there is *NOTHING*..

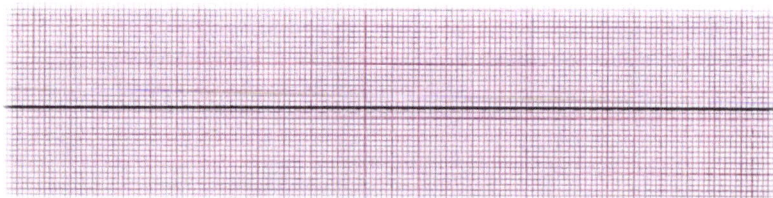

www.ingramcontent.com/pod-product-compliance
Lightning Source LLC
Chambersburg PA
CBHW040305220526
45473CB00002B/587

Understanding ECGs has never been easier than with ECGs Made Easy..

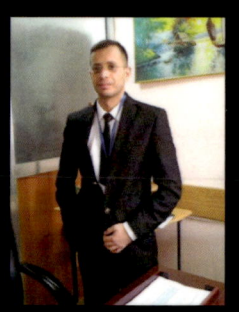

THIS book represents the first STEPs to ECG interpretation , that should you have !!